D1325386

Stay Healthy.
Be Lazy.

an easy detox by innocent

published by Boxtree

First published 2004 by Boxtree.
An imprint of Pan Macmillan, 20 New Wharf Road, London N1 9RR
Basingstoke, Oxford and associated companies throughout the world.
www.panmacmillan.com

ISBN-13: 978-0-7522-1595-0
ISBN-10: 0-7522-1595-7

A CIP catalogue record for this book is available from the British Library.

Printed by Proost, Belgium.

Hello mum.

Contents

Hello

We thought we'd start off by saying why we wrote this book. And really, it's the same reason that we started making smoothies — to make it a bit easier to do yourself some good.

We all know how to be healthy — drink less beer, eat your greens, cycle to work. But then we forget it all and eat family size bags of Cheezi Num-Nums for breakfast. So the purpose of this book is to remind you about the stuff you already know, to introduce you to some new ideas and to incorporate some healthy habits into your life without turning you into a health freak.

To help us make all of this delox stuff a bit easier, we turned to the experts. Our friend Professor Joe Millward made sure we were getting all of the food and drink bits right, whilst Pete Williams, personal trainer to the stars (and nice normal people too), gave us lots of ideas and info on every aspect of exercise.

And after listening to them and getting all of the information together in one place, it became pretty clear to us. If you read this book and follow the advice contained within, we reckon you'll be a lot healthier and happier. If you already do all of this stuff, then we salute you – you can skip the words and just look at the pictures. But if you're like us (i.e. lazy), this little refresher course in being nice to your body should go down a treat.

How to use this book

We've split the book into seven sections, the idea being that you read a section a day (on the bus, before you go to bed) and learn a few new things. At the end of each section there are the three golden rules, so if you can't be bothered to read the whole book, then at least read those bits.

What we hope is that by the time you've finished the book, enough of the ideas will have lodged in your brain that you'll start to incorporate them into your everyday life without it being too much effort. And you can keep referring back for new ideas and exercises when you get bored of the old ones.

What is detoxing?

People seem to overuse and misuse the word 'detox' these days. But what it basically means is...

If you are constantly boozing, smoking and eating rubbish, your liver (the organ that processes nasty toxins) gets overworked and doesn't have time to get rid of all of those toxins, meaning that they build up elsewhere in your body. In essence, detoxing is laying off the bad stuff and eating and drinking well for a while, which gives the liver time to process the backlog of toxins stored in your body.

Obviously this is a simplified description, but if you drink enough water, try to have a relatively healthy diet and do a bit of exercise, you'll be helping your body to process the odd few bad things that come your way on a rolling basis, without having to set aside special 'detox time'.

In other words, we say that your whole life can be one long easy detox, doing away with the need to stick a hosepipe up your bum and drink cabbage water three times a day.

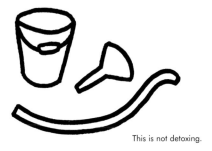

This is not detoxing.

day one

drink water

You are
70% water

So am I, and so is that man over there.
We were going to start a Water Fan Club for the three of us,
but then we thought it would be better if we talked about it in
this book. We're starting off with water because it's the most
important thing we put into our bodies. Every time we breathe
or blink or twitch, we are using up water in the shape of one
bodily process or another, and as we have no way of storing
water, we need to top up our supplies constantly.

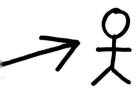

Water does some very important things in order to make our bodies work properly. It ferries away waste products through the kidneys in the form of urine, scientifically known as wee*.
It helps to move nutrients around our bodies, and most of the vital chemical reactions within our cells occur in water. Your brain is about 75% water, so when you're trying to do a very difficult sum, it often helps to have a sip or two. And if you're properly hydrated, you'll have more energy, as your body will be able to convert fat into usable energy.

*If you want to find out more about the science of weeing, take a look at the back flap of this book.

The water cycle

We thought we'd put this here to show that we remembered some stuff from school. And because it's one of nature's best tricks; moving water without buckets.

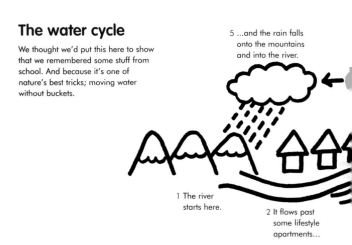

5 ...and the rain falls onto the mountains and into the river.

1 The river starts here.

2 It flows past some lifestyle apartments...

The health of your skin is also reliant on a good and constant supply of water. The skin is one of the body's major organs and needs water to maintain the health of its cells. Unfortunately, other organs, such as the brain, take precedence when it comes to the allocation of water supplies, which means that if you aren't getting enough water, your skin will be one of the first things to suffer.

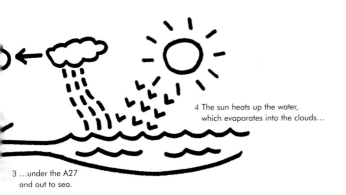

4 The sun heats up the water,
  which evaporates into the clouds...

3 ...under the A27
  and out to sea.

So without water, we would quite simply fall apart, making it very difficult to go to the shops or get on the train to visit your favourite aunt out in the country. But if you make sure that you are drinking enough, then your body will be working efficiently and effectively.

So how much water should you drink?

A lot of the water that your body needs is obtained from food, especially fruit and veg. But you definitely need a separate intake of water as well. And the Department of Health advises adults to drink at least 6-8 cups or glasses a day, which works out to be about 2 litres*.

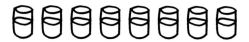

Your daily intake of water should look something like this.

Of course, there are some circumstances under which your body might ask for a bit more – for instance, if you are breast-feeding, if you live somewhere hot (chance would be a fine thing), or if you're recovering from illness.

*If you have been hiding in a cupboard since drinking some of the spiked punch at that *Sergeant Pepper* album launch party, 2 litres is a bit less than 4 pints.

What about if I exercise lots?

If you exercise regularly, you should increase the amount of water you drink. Ideally, drink an extra glass or two before exercising (not directly before, unless you like the sound of sloshing) as well as some afterwards.

The following chart shows the number of extra glasses of water you should drink per day according to how hard you exercise. Feel the burn.

Your weight (kg)	One hour of light activity e.g. walking	One hour of moderate activity e.g. a gentle jog	One hour of strenuous activity e.g. a full sweaty workout
50	1	2	3
60	1	2	3
70	1	2	3
80	2	2	4
90	2	3	4
100*	3	4	5

*This one's for Alan Valon.

How can I make sure I drink my 2 litres every day?

If you are one of those people who just doesn't like water, or you're just a bit lazy, there are all sorts of ways in which you can make it easier to get your daily intake, and make it more palatable too.

Add a splash of fruit juice or a slice of lemon or lime to a glass of water.

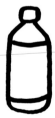

Fill up a 2-litre bottle when you get to work, stick it on your desk and don't go home until it's finished.

Drink hot water with a bit of lemon or ginger instead of tea or coffee.

Walk around with your mouth open when it's raining.

How about a nice cup of tea?

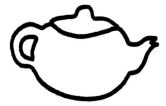

There's nothing better than a nice cup of tea, apart from maybe winning a game of naked darts against that special someone. And because tea is seen as a remedy for everything from heartbreak to post-traffic accident shock, you might think that it would be a good idea to get your daily intake of water with a drop of milk and two sugars.

Unfortunately that's not the case, and this goes for coffee, fizzy pop and beer too, all of which mostly consist of water. They don't count. When we talk about 2 litres of water, we're talking about 2 litres of straight, pure water on top of the other things that you drink and eat. Your body needs it to help process the gunk in the other things that you consume. So please help it.

Having said that, it's better to drink tea than no liquid at all, but drinks like tea, coffee and cola contain caffeine, which is a diuretic. This means that they will make you wee, which means that you'll need even more water just to replace the wee.

If you're still desperate for a brew, our friend David is quite particular about how to make a nice cup of tea. Here are his full instructions for making a nice drop:

1. Boil fresh water.
2. Warm the pot and the cups.
3. Place one rounded teaspoon of tea per person in the pot.
4. As soon as the kettle has boiled pour the water on the leaves and stir.
5. Leave for 3-4 minutes, depending on how strong you like it.
6. Add milk first to your cup.
7. Pour tea when ready.
8. Phew.

by David Hieatt
H.O.T (Head of Tea) and co-founder of Cardigan Bay's third biggest clothing company. Visit www.howies.co.uk which is where David lives.

So which kind of water is best?

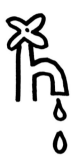

Tap

In the UK it is accepted that tap water is safe to drink, so there is seemingly no reason why you shouldn't get your recommended daily allowance (RDA) the cheap way. But many people argue that tap water contains nitrates, or heavy metals such as lead and aluminium, which don't do you any good. However, it should be stressed that in 2001, water companies in England and Wales carried out approximately 2.8 million tests on drinking water samples of which 99.86% passed. If you're really concerned, get information from your local water company or check out the Drinking Water Inspectorate website – www.dwi.gov.uk, the people who make sure your tap water is fit to drink.

Filtered

Makers of filter jugs agree that tap water in the UK is safe. But they sell their filter jugs on the premise that tap water still contains impurities that might not make it taste or smell so good. Their filters will reduce the amount of such things as chlorine (used to disinfect our water supply), magnesium and calcium (both of which cause hard water and fur up your kettle), and heavy metals (such as lead, which usually comes from old water pipes).

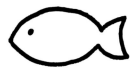

Fish are born with efficient water filtration systems, known as gills. Apart from in *The Man from Atlantis*, this has never happened to a human, leading us to buy filter jugs instead.

Bottled

There are two main types of bottled water – natural mineral water and spring water. By definition, both must be extracted from an underground source. But where they differ is as follows:

Natural mineral water should have a constant mineral content. And it can't be treated, except to filter out grit, or to remove 'unstable elements' such as iron, which can discolour the water. There are no limits on the maximum levels of 'good' minerals such as calcium and potassium.

Spring water can have a variable mineral content. It has to meet the same hygiene standards as natural mineral water, and is subject to the same limits on pollution. But, unlike natural mineral water, UK-produced spring water can be treated so that it reaches these standards.

So on the face of it, natural mineral water can be more 'natural' than spring water, as it might contain more good minerals and is untreated. But there isn't that much difference.

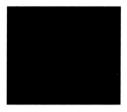

The view from inside
a spring water well.

What we reckon

Firstly, we reckon it's all quite confusing. But it's worth thinking about, seeing as water is the most important stuff that we put in our bodies. Our conclusion is that we want you to drink lots of water, so you should do it by drinking whichever type of water you find most convenient, or choose the one that appeals most to your tastebuds or wallet. They're all safe, and they all taste of water.

In a nutshell

1 drink 2 litres of water a day

2 don't worry about where it comes from – tap, mineral and filter are all fine

3 too much tea and coffee will ruin all of your water-drinking hard work, so try to limit your brews

eat some fruit and veg

What's so good about fruit and veg?

We all know that fruit and veg are very good stuff. The NHS advises that the second most important thing you can do to reduce the risk of cancer and heart disease is to eat more fruit and veg (the first is not to smoke). What's more, fruit and veg actually taste nice, look good in your kitchen and contain all of the vital nutrients that you need for a healthy life; the stuff that your body just can't make itself.

So our advice to you, always and forever, is that if you want to do one thing to make your life happier and healthier, eat lots of fruit and veg. The next few pages explain how to make sure you do it, with lots of recipes and some essential information about allotments right at the end.

So what are the bits in fruit and veg that are good for you?

Most of the good things in fruit and veg are known as phytoprotectants, an umbrella term for just about all of the natural nutrients you'll find in your average apple or cabbage. Phytoprotectants include things like antioxidants (vitamins A, C, E, carotenoids, selenium, etc), which keep your cells healthy, your immune system strong, your eyes blessed with vision...everything really. Fruit and veg also contain minerals, such as folate and potassium, which keep your blood strong and your heart and muscles in good nick. The following pages tell you how much fruit and veg you need so you can get the right amounts of all of these good things in your diet, naturally.

29

How much fruit and veg should I eat each day?

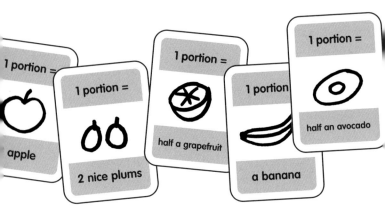

1 portion =

apple

1 portion =

2 nice plums

1 portion =

half a grapefruit

1 portion

a banana

1 portion =

half an avocado

Five a day is a message that you've probably got quite bored of hearing, but it's the main thing as far as fruit and veg are concerned. Please eat five portions a day. And remember that it's a minimum, so it won't hurt to eat more.

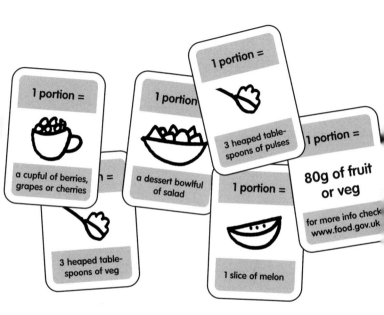

1 portion =

a cupful of berries, grapes or cherries

1 portion =

a dessert bowlful of salad

1 portion =

3 heaped table-spoons of pulses

1 portion =

80g of fruit or veg

for more info check www.food.gov.uk

1 portion =

3 heaped table-spoons of veg

1 portion =

1 slice of melon

Naturally, fresh is best, but dried, tinned or frozen will do just fine. And variety is key too – eating fruit and veg of different colours and textures means you'll get a wider range of nutrients into your diet. So it's no good eating five bananas before you nip down to the Dog and Trumpet for ladies' darts night.

How lazy people can still eat lots of fruit and veg

"But I'm busy. I haven't got time to prepare three different vegetables every evening when I get home after a hard day in my swivel chair."

We hear you. Sometimes you just can't be bothered. And modern life can make things difficult – we work longer hours, live further away from work and have loads more things to distract us from the noble art of cooking vegetables and eating fruit. So here are some tips to make getting your five a day as painless and natural as possible.

Why fruit and veg are better than pills

It is a scientific fact that the stuff that comes in peel and skin is better for you than the stuff that comes in little brown bottles. Obviously it would be great if you could get a little manmade pill that provided all of the benefits of a diet rich in fruit and veg. But it isn't going to happen, and anyone who tells you otherwise is probably trying to sell you some pills.

Meals

Never let a meal time go by without taking the opportunity to contribute something to your five a day...

- Breakfast – stick a banana on your cornflakes or some fresh berries in your Cheerios. Dried cranberries work well on just about anything.

- Lunch – if you're having a sandwich, make sure it's got salad and tomatoes in it. Or maybe even some avocado. And have some grapes or a tangerine instead of that Penguin.

- Dinner – chuck beans and bits of apple in your curry, use fresh toms and peas in your pasta sauce, and, if you're lazy, buy bags of that pre-chopped salad.

These are little ideas, but there are some recipes starting on page 45 that make getting your 5 a day even easier and tastier.

Snacks

We like snacks. They help fill the time between meals quite nicely, and, if you do them right, you can knock a few of your five a day on the head during morning and afternoon break.

- Choose fruit salad instead of crisps, or a nice bag of cherries instead of that Wagon Wheel.

- Packets of dried fruit on your desk are a good idea. They don't go off so you can keep them there for a while.

- If you're prepared, have some fruit and veg chopped up in your lunch box – carrot sticks, tomato wedges, sliced up bits of pineapple, mango...

Crisps. Tasty, but a bit rubbish.

Drinks

You can mash, blend and juice your fruit and veg to make juices and smoothies (this amazing insight has served us well over the last few years).

- Buy your favourite fruit and veg and make up a big smoothie in the morning. Drink a bit, take the rest to work and feel free to chug throughout the day.

- Impress your friends. Get a fancy blender for your kitchen.

- Or get your boss to buy a blender for the kitchen at work – a healthy workforce is a happy workforce.

- If you're a bit lazy like us, buy a smoothie that someone else has put into a bottle for you. Ours contain your recommended daily intake of fruit, which makes it all quite easy.

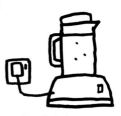

It s like a kettle for the new millennium.

When you're out

There are plenty of places to get fruit and veg while you're down the shops buying lampshades and tennis balls.

- Good sandwich shops sell decent salads which will take care of a portion of veg.

- And don't forget fruit stalls, greengrocers and your local market.

- If you're in KFC, go for the sweetcorn and beans.

- McDonald's now sell little bags of fruit that count as one of your five a day portions, and Boots sell nice packets of carrot sticks.

Getting kids to eat more fruit and veg

Good food helps your children grow up big and strong, so here are some ideas to stop them from subsisting solely on a diet of cheese strings and pizza nuggets.

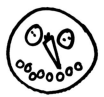

- You may mock, but drawing a funny face with veg on a dinner plate will encourage consumption.

- Make ice lollies from nice fresh fruit juice.

- When making jelly, chuck in some fresh fruit before it has set.

- Stick dried fruit in their lunch boxes.

- And don't say, "If you eat all your veg you can have lots of chocolate." You'll just be asking for it.

Fresh vs frozen

Fresh veg is great, but then so is frozen stuff. In fact, some frozen stuff will contain more nutrients as it was frozen at source and not transported halfway across the world in its natural state. Keep it in your freezer and throw in a handful whenever you are making pasta/risotto/veg surprise. Like we said before, fresh, frozen or tinned – it's all good.

Prepared vs not

If buying bags of pre-washed and chopped veg and salad means that you'll eat it, then please do it. It may cost a few pence more, but if it's going to make it easier for you to get involved then it's money well spent. And if you're going to buy ready meals, get some with veg in them. Chicken sag is much better for you than chicken korma. The same goes for pasta – choose spinach or tomato sauces over creamy ones.

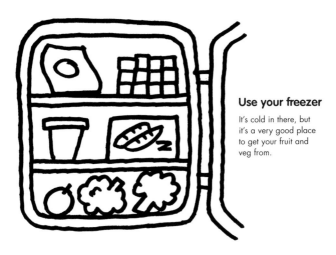

Use your freezer

It's cold in there, but it's a very good place to get your fruit and veg from.

Organic or not?

The organic debate is developing and changing all of the time. So what you're getting is what we thought when we wrote this book. We reserve the right to develop and change our minds, but at the moment...if the concept of eating organically makes it more likely that you'll get your five a day, then great. Anything that encourages people to do this is a good thing. But we don't think that an absence of organic produce should stop you from eating fruit and veg. And eating organic doughnuts and drinking organic vodka doesn't make you more healthy.

Top ten fruit and veg

(a bit like *Top of the Pops*, but with carrots instead of the Sugababes)

Here are the best fruit and veg in the world. In our opinion. Apologies to the ones we left out. Maybe next time?

 Blueberries ...contain more antioxidant power than broccoli, spinach or garlic, which means that they help in the fight against cancer, ageing and heart disease.

 Bananas ...provide potassium for energy and a healthy ticker. They also contain the eight essential amino acids, which are crucial for building healthy cells.

 Cranberries ...having a good wee is always a pleasure, especially if you've been waiting all the way since junction 19. Cranberries make weeing healthier, killing bacteria and viruses in the urinary tract.

 Apples ...contain pectin, which helps to remove heavy metals from your body, such as the lead that you breathe in via traffic fumes.

Tomatoes …are 90% water, so help to keep you hydrated. They also contain lycopene, a powerful antioxidant thought to help prevent prostate cancer.

 Lemons and limes …squeeze them over your salad or fish or veg to make them taste all fresh and exotic. They're full of vitamin C and potassium.

 Spinach …is green and tasty. And it's full of iron, folic acid, beta-carotene, helps to shore up your immune system and makes you dead tough.

 Mangoes …the pinky-orange colour of mango flesh is a sign that it's rich in beta-carotene, which the body turns into vitamin A, essential for healthy skin and eyes.

 Carrots …contain carotenoids, which will help the body battle against asthma, heart disease, cancer and arthritis.

 Broccoli …is full of fibre, vitamin C and loads of other antioxidants. Tastes lovely too.

an ode to broccoli

Shall I compare thee to a summer's day?
Or perhaps a lump of broccoli?
Sprouting florets of goodness
And looking a bit like a cauliflower

For it is you that my heart desires
Because all of those vitamins
Will surely make me healthy and wise
And you're very nice with rice and fish

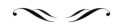

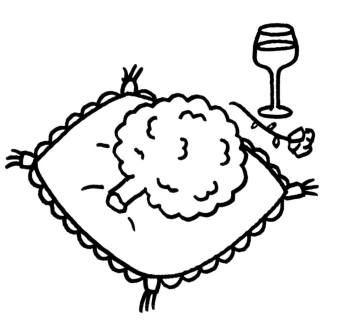

Steam it

Cooking doesn't mean boiling stuff while you go off to watch *The Godfather* box set on DVD. The longer you cook fruit and veg, the more it becomes a nutrition-free mush. So invest in a steamer. Steaming uses less water, makes the veg taste nicer and is the best way to cook if you're interested in getting the maximum nutritional benefits. Those bamboo ones are dead cheap and can be worn as a hat if you're searching for a new look.

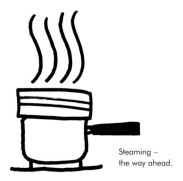

Steaming –
the way ahead.

Fruit and veg recipes

Here are some recipes that we've made up, borrowed from friends and begged from some very clever and able chefs.

Space precludes us from printing millions of them, but you should be able to get more good ideas from any decent cookbook, or just from your mum.

Our patented Portion Trump Card™
is displayed next to each recipe,
showing you how many fruit and/or
veg portions the dish provides
per person.

Unless stated otherwise, all recipes serve four people.

Our famous purple detox smoothie

The nice thing about this is that it's not like you have to force yourself to drink it. It contains blueberries (the fruit world's richest source of antioxidants), it's very tasty and it comes up a beautiful shade of mauve.

Ingredients

- 1 pineapple
- 1 handful of blueberries (about 30 or so)
- The juice of 1 orange (to make it runny enough to drink)

What to do

- Plug your blender in.

- Chop up the pineapple into small chunks (big chunks don't blend so easily).

- Pop into the blender with the other ingredients and blitz.

- Drink it all up and scrape out the jug with a spoon.

fruit/veg

2

portions

Assia's anti-asthma smoothie

Our Assia gets asthma bad. So her nice boyfriend Steve invented this for her. He says it helps because of the quercetin and bromelain (found in apples and pineapples respectively), which work well together as natural anti-inflammatory agents, helping to calm her lungs. Sounds scientific, tastes f-f-fresh.

Ingredients

- 1 pear
- 2 apples
- 2 radishes or horseradishes
- 20 baby spinach leaves
- 1 pineapple
- 2 large carrots
- 2 bananas
- The juice of 1 lemon
- 2 cloves of garlic (optional but very good for you)

What to do

- Juice the pear, apples, radishes, spinach, pineapple and carrots.

- Add all of this juice to your blender with the bananas, lemon juice (and garlic if you're feeling lucky).

- Whizz it up, drink and feel the power.

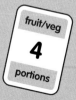

fruit/veg

4

portions

Grape, rocket and Parmesan salad

This one is very simple, sounds quite posh and is oh-so-easy to stick in a bowl in the morning to take to work. Remember, a bowl of salad knocks one of your five portions on the head, so it's worth making and eating.

Ingredients

- 4 handfuls of rocket
- 2 handfuls of grapes
- Some thin shavings of Parmesan

For the dressing

- Black pepper
- A drizzle of extra virgin olive oil
- A squeeze of lemon

What to do

• Wash your leaves and grapes.

• Stick them in a bowl and dress with the Parmesan and dressing.

• Make fashionable chit-chat whilst eating, just as you would in a posh restaurant. Mentioning your new cottage in rural Wiltshire or that new Ann Demeulemeester frock will do for starters.

fruit/veg

1

portions

Shrimp and citrus martini

A prawn cocktail for people who like *Sex and the City*. And it's stuffed with fruit. One to impress the neighbours with, if you are ever brave enough to invite them round for dinner.

Ingredients

- 300g of nice fat tiger prawns, chopped into chunks
- 1 orange, peeled, de-pithed, segmented and cut into small chunks
- 1 grapefruit, as above
- 1 red onion, finely sliced
- 1 tsp chives, chopped
- 1 avocado, finely diced
- Some chives to make it look pretty

What to do

- Mix all ingredients together, apart from the avocado and a few unchopped chives, which you should save to put on the top.

- Season with salt and pepper.

- Assemble everything in martini glasses, top with the avocado and chives, chill in the fridge for a few minutes and, like, serve.

fruit/veg

4

portions

Nigel's grilled antipasto

In return for a box of smoothies and a bag of chips, that nice Nigel Slater gave us a recipe to use. It's from his book *Appetite*.

Ingredients

- 4 red peppers, halved
- Olive oil
- 2 big aubergines
- A couple of handfuls of herbs – mainly basil, with a bit of fresh oregano and flat leaf parsley, all torn up
- 4 cloves of garlic, thinly sliced
- Lemon – to squeeze

What to do

- Stick the halved peppers in a baking tin with a splash of olive oil and bake at 200°C/Gas 6 till they are soft (30-50 minutes). Leave them to cool before taking out the seeds and removing the skin.

- While the peppers are cooking, slice the aubergine about as thick as your little finger, brush with oil and a bit of salt, and pop them in a ridged grill pan on a moderate heat.

- Cook on each side till they are golden-brown and have those fancy deep black lines etched on them from the pan. Check they are cooked right through before removing them.

- Mix the aubergines, peppers, herbs, garlic, good olive oil, lemon juice and seasoning in a bowl.

- Let it all cool to room temperature before serving with some good bread and stuff.

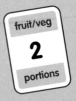

fruit/veg

2

portions

Mango salsa

Let's face it – that salsa you buy in jars to stick corn chips into is a bit old hat. Here's our fruit-based alternative, which not only serves as a dip but also as a nice thing to eat with barbecued or grilled fish and meat.

Ingredients

- 2 ripe medium-sized mangoes, finely diced
- 250g of cherry tomatoes, chopped
- 4 spring onions, chopped
- A small handful of coriander, chopped
- The juice of a lime
- Salt and pepper

What to do

• Mix all of the ingredients together in a big bowl.

• Invite your friends over and eat the dip just like on the advert.

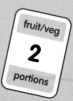

fruit/veg

2

portions

Beetroot risotto

Something warm and filling for a winter's night. Our Lucy says to wear rubber gloves to stop you from getting pink hands.

Ingredients

- Olive oil
- 1 small onion, chopped
- 2 garlic cloves, chopped
- 3 medium raw beetroot, peeled and very thinly sliced
- 400g of risotto rice
- 125ml of white wine
- 500g of passata
- 1 litre of veg stock
- Soft goat's cheese
- Basil leaves, torn up

What to do

• Using a big saucepan, soften the onion in the oil over a low heat. Add the garlic and beetroot and cook for 4-5 minutes, stirring occasionally.

• Stir in the rice, letting it soak up the juices. Then add the wine, stirring all the time. Once the rice has soaked up the wine, stir in the passata. Simmer for 3-4 minutes until most of the liquid has been absorbed.

• Pour one quarter of the stock into the pan. Simmer gently, stirring until the excess liquid has been absorbed.

• Continue adding the stock a splash at a time, stirring and letting the rice soak it up, until the rice is tender but has a slight bite – should take about 25-30 minutes. Don't worry if it's still slightly gooey – that's how it should be.

• Stir in your crumbled goat's cheese and basil at the end and serve on white plates for maximum redness.

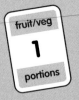

fruit/veg

1

portions

Clare's quick Thai sweet potato curry

Clare is a special girl with a special recipe.

Ingredients

- 5 or 6 medium sized sweet potatoes, peeled and cut into chunks
- The grated zest and juice of 2 limes
- Groundnut oil (olive oil will do though)
- 2 green chillis, chopped (de-seed them if you don't like it hot)
- A tin of half-fat coconut milk
- 2 handfuls of coriander leaves, chopped roughly
- 8 spring onions, chopped
- Soy or fish sauce
- 2 heads of pak choi, torn up, or a couple of handfuls of baby leaf spinach
- Enough rice or noodles for four

What to do

• Parboil the sweet potatoes till they begin to soften. Drain them and then marinate in the lime juice and zest for half an hour. Get everything else ready while they soak up the lime.

• Heat a drop of oil in your wok and stick the potatoes, lime juice and zest in for a minute, stirring all the time. Add the chopped chillies and stir for half a minute.

• Add the coconut milk, half the coriander and half the spring onions. Then cook for another couple of minutes, have a taste and season with a drop of soy sauce, or fish sauce to remain truly authentic.

• Turn off the heat and stir in your pak choi or spinach. You just want to wilt this a little, rather than cook it.

• Serve with rice or noodles and the rest of the spring onions and coriander on top, which Clare reckons makes it look dead posh.

fruit/veg

2

portions

Kylie's apricot cake

All the way from Perth, Western Australia, tested on generations of our Kylie's family, this is a fat-free fruit-filled cake. She swears by it, and so does her gran.

Ingredients

- 375g of mixed dried fruit
- 450g of tinned apricots that you purée, juice and all
- 125g of self-raising flour

What to do

- Soak the dried fruit in the apricot mush overnight in a covered container in the fridge.

- Next day, mix in the flour.

- Put it all into a 25cm loaf tin and bake for 1-1/2 hours at about 180°C.

- Let it cool, stick it in a padded envelope and send it to Kylie's gran for an independent assessment.

fruit/veg

2

portions

Cheese and biscuits

We love cheese, so it would be a shame to leave it out altogether, although we don't recommend it for pudding every night.

Ingredients

- Lots of cheese
- The fruit of your choice
- Biscuits (oatcakes are very good for you)

What to do

• An hour or two before eating the cheese, unwrap it and leave it to acclimatise at room temperature.

• When you're ready, serve the cheese with your favourite fruits – apples, grapes, figs, pears...

• Eat your cheese and fruit with the oatcakes.

• Finished the cheese? Then it's time to retire to the drawing room for brandy, cigars and stimulating chats about the markets.

Depends on how much fruit you eat with your cheese.

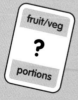

fruit/veg

?

portions

Grow your own

There's nothing like growing your own fruit and veg. But if you don't have a garden, you might want to find out about getting an allotment. According to Geoff at the National Society of Allotment and Leisure Gardeners, an allotment is capable of producing £500 worth of produce a year, enough to feed a family of four.

To get one, phone your local council, ask for the person in charge of allotments and see if they have any that are up for grabs. They're usually dead cheap – the average rent is £25 per year, but it does vary from as little as £3 to £70 depending on the area and facilities.

When you think about it, what you're doing is maintaining spare land for your council, so it should be cheap. And here's a good thing – if six or more people put in a request, your council is legally obliged to find an allotment site for you.

Thanks to Geoff Stokes at the National Society of Allotment and Leisure Gardeners
www.nsalg.org.uk or www.nsalg.demon.co.uk

In other words

1 get your five a day
   however you can – fresh,
   frozen, tinned, steamed...

2 don't rely on pills to do
   nature's job

3 marry a lump of broccoli

get a balanced diet

Why bother eating well?

We don't know about you, but eating good food makes us very excited. It's a sensory pleasure, just like listening to great music or gazing at a beautiful landscape. But before we get too misty-eyed about the contents of our fridge, it's worth explaining exactly why it's worth eating well. As if you didn't know…

If you want to be healthy, you should have a diet that includes all of the different food groups – things like carbohydrates, protein, vitamins, minerals and fats (more about them in the next few pages). Eating such a diet means you'll have more energy during the day, you'll sleep better at night, your mind will be sharper, your breath sweeter and your eyes just a little more twinklier*.

*This is a new word, we hope you enjoy it.

The opposite obviously applies – if you stuff your face with rubbish whenever you fancy, your body won't like you very much, your brain won't be getting all of the fuel it needs, and you could feel pretty miserable.

Special diets that cut out entire food groups are no good either. All they do is omit nutrients that are necessary to keep your body healthy and strong forever. Long term, this will affect you both physically and mentally, whereas a proper balanced diet will make you feel fighting fit and will also help you to feel balanced emotionally.

So in this section we'll try to help you eat the right sort of stuff, without having to sacrifice all of the things that you really like.

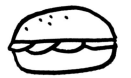

There are only three things that are certain in this life: death, taxes and cheese rolls.

What makes up a balanced diet?

There's no mystery to the balanced diet – it's all about eating the right amounts of different types of food. And everyone knows what that entails – more fruit and veg, more high-fibre foods, less saturated fats and less processed stuff. But there are differing opinions over what proportions of certain foods we should eat. And it's all about the food groups.

So what are the food groups?

We discuss these in a bit more depth in the following pages, but foods generally fall into three different areas:

• Carbohydrates to give you energy.

• Protein to help the body build and repair itself.

• Fats, which can be both good and bad (more details later).

How much of all of this stuff should I eat then?

In the UK we have nutrient recommendations for two of the three main areas – <35% fat and 10% protein, leaving 55% for carbohydrates. But some people argue for a 30:10:60 split. General guidelines are given on the Food Standards Agency's website www.food.gov.uk.

There's also www.nal.usda.gov/fnic/Fpyr/pymid.gif, where you can see the US food pyramid, which gives servings per day for the main food groups.

Generally, food-based dietary guidelines are poorly developed in the UK, so have a look at the above and read what follows over the next few pages to work out what's good for you. After all of that you should be ready for a lie-down and a chocolate digestive.

We got lots of this information from Professor Joe Millward, Director of the Centre for Food Safety and Nutrition at the University of Surrey, a world-leading authority on human nutrition, an adviser to the UK government and an all-round lovely man.

Carbohydrates and energy

Carbs provide fuel to power the body. The body breaks them down into glucose (our primary source of energy), which is absorbed into the bloodstream and carried away by insulin to the body's muscle and liver cells, where it can get to work.

However (and this is the dull but important bit), there are good carbs and bad carbs. What sets them apart is their 'glycaemic index' (GI) – a fancy name for the measure of how quickly carbs take to break down and enter the blood stream. 'Good' carbs have a low GI i.e. they take longer to break down and therefore provide a more constant, slow-release energy supply.

But carbs with a high GI break down quickly, causing the amount of glucose in the blood stream (blood sugar level) to rise quickly. This is bad because the body can't cope with it all, and so calls upon insulin to remove the glucose and store it as fat. Disappointing. Furthermore, because this leaves the blood almost empty of glucose, our brains tell us that it's time to get more energy. So our instinct is to eat rubbish sugary food to get instant energy, thus completing a vicious circle.

The bottom line is that if you want to avoid unnecessary weight gain, stay away from bad, cheap carbs and eat good carbs with a low GI. Or to put it another way, lose the doughnuts.

Eat more of these	Eat less of these
Lower GI = slow release energy	Higher GI = quick release energy
Wholemeal and rye bread	White bread
Wholemeal pasta and noodles	White pasta
Brown rice	White rice
Couscous	Nights in white satin
Yoghurt	Parsnips
Sweet potatoes	Old brown bananas
Soya beans (tofu etc)	Carrots (cooked)
Carrots (raw)	Fizzy sugary pop
Brazil nuts and almonds	Sweets
Chick peas and lentils	Chocolate
Just about all fruit	
Oatcakes	

Bananas are special, changing from low to high GI when ripening, so don't wait until they get brown. Eat the ones with green tips (not too green or you might not feel so good). Cold boiled spuds are good too – they have a low GI, as opposed to ones that are still hot, which have a high GI. So eat potato salad (easy on the mayo).

Protein

You're not the same person you used to be. Or to put it another way, the body regenerates its cells every six months. And as proteins are the building blocks that make up everything from the collagen that keeps your skin looking nice, to the antibodies in your blood that keep disease at bay, you need them to help build a stronger, better you all of the time.

As for good places to get lots of protein from, meat and eggs are rich sources, but nuts, seeds, cheese, beans, pulses and soya all contain protein. So vegetarians needn't go without.

Protein performs another important function – it helps to manage your energy levels. It does this by slowing down the digestive process, simply because it takes a bit longer to digest. Consequently, blood sugar levels don't rise so sharply, so energy will be released more steadily. Make sure that when consuming large amounts of carbs at lunch or dinner, you also temper them with some protein.

Fats

People get a bit freaked about fat. But you shouldn't be trying to cut it out of your diet — just cut your consumption of bad fats.

Bad fat — the fats that aren't good for you tend to be solid at room temperature, like butter, cheese and the crispy bits attached to your bacon. They fur up arteries and are generally bad, especially for your heart and your trousers. Sometimes referred to as saturated or animal fats.

Good fat — these are liquid at room temperature; sources include olive, fish and nut oils, as well as green veg, oily fish and fresh nuts and seeds themselves. Essential fatty acids (EFAs) found in good fats are thought to help lower cholesterol, help you lose weight and aid in the fight against heart disease and cancer. And the omega 3 oils found in oily fish help to prevent heart disease and the onset of Alzheimer's, so eat up all of your mackerel and smoked salmon.

It should be noted that heating good fats such as olive oil knocks out the good bits of the EFAs, so to get the goodness, don't heat them.

Vitamins and minerals

Vitamins are a group of organic compounds that are needed in minute amounts for growth and good health. They ensure that just about every bodily function is working well and properly, from the immune system to strong bones to healthy skin to good eyesight. If you eat a healthy, balanced, natural diet, you'll be getting all of the vitamins you need. Therefore, we don't think that you need to take supplements (see page 32) unless it's for a medical reason.

The same goes for minerals – a healthy diet means you'll be getting all that you need. Minerals are good for healthy blood, strong bones and teeth, and for converting food into energy. You get minerals from dark green veg, dairy stuff, meat, pulses, eggs, dried fruit – everything really.

A good source of information is www.food.gov.uk, the website of the Food Standards Agency.

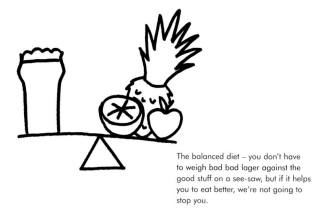

The balanced diet – you don't have to weigh bad bad lager against the good stuff on a see-saw, but if it helps you to eat better, we're not going to stop you.

What we reckon

The thing we've noticed, being dead observant and everything, is that if you are getting a good mix of all of these important food groups, you'll be a lot healthier. And if you eat cheese on toast three times a day you are in trouble. But never fear – over the page we suggest a very nice healthy balanced menu that should sort you out.

So what do I eat to get a balanced diet?

Here's an ideal menu. We're sure you've seen this kind of thing before; whether or not you actually followed it to the letter is another matter.

But we put it here to highlight a couple of things. Firstly, it's pretty painless, and full of tasty food. Secondly, there are no weird, faddish foods – they're all the sort of things that we know are good for us. We just want to show that normal people with normal fridges and normal cravings for chips and gravy can eat the right stuff too.

Just go easy on the chips and gravy.

Homemade houmous saves you cash and tastes lovely. Stick lots of drained and rinsed tinned chick peas, virgin olive oil, lemon juice and cumin into a bowl and mash them all up, or whizz them in your blender. Easy enough even for the laziest person. Keeps for a couple of days in the fridge.

an ideal menu

Breakfast
Eggs (poached or boiled) on wholemeal toast.
or
Muesli or porridge (not Ready Brek) with fresh fruit on top.

Morning break
Nice fresh fruit, and maybe some unsalted nuts and seeds.

Lunchtime
Wholemeal chicken sandwich with salad (hold the mayo).

Afternoon snack
A Penguin (oops).

Dinner/tea/whatever you call it
A nice bit of fish (not from the chip shop), lots of steamed veg
and a couple of glasses of wine for being so good today.

How to make
the perfect packed lunch

My best packed lunch at school used to be meat-paste sandwiches (on Mighty White) with a packet of cheese and onion and a Blue Riband. Unfortunately, even though this is a timeless classic, it's not going to make you any healthier. So here is a packed lunch to make you healthy. And it tastes nice too.

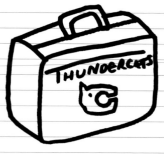

my favourite
Thundercats
lunchbox

Build layers of these in your favourite big tupperware:

★ cooked brown rice or wholemeal noodles
★ a can of good beans like cannelini or kidney beans
★ a can of tuna, or some cooked fresh fish if you've got some, you posh thing
★ lots of chopped veg (salad stuff, tomatoes, green beans, mange tout etc)
★ a generous drop of extra virgin olive oil and some of your favourite vinegar
★ lots of seeds and nuts on the top

It's a bit like your very own bespoke salad niçoise in a tub. And you can use other ingredients too – grilled chicken, boiled eggs and any veg you can think of. Stick it all in the tub before you go to bed, put it in the fridge and the next day you'll be the envy of your meat-paste-sandwich-eating colleagues (as long as you remember to get it out of the fridge and take it to work).

9/10 ✓

What to eat when

It's not always easy to know what to eat at particular times. So here are some practical and reasonable suggestions for things to eat when faced with certain situations...

...when you are drunk

Logic is not a good guide in the land of the merry sailor. But please try to avoid fried stuff like the plague – choose tandoori chicken, and plain rice instead of special fried. If you end up in Idaho Fried Chicken, go for the grilled chicken and the beans.

...when you are hungover

Steer clear of processed and fried foods, which just overload your liver when it's already working overtime. Help it by drinking lots of warm water with fresh lemon in it. Avoid alcohol, coffee or tea, and be sure to eat unprocessed foods – brown toast is good.

...when you are feeling low

Wholegrain foods such as brown rice, rye and barley contain B vitamins, which help lift your mood. Eggs and oily fish are good sources too. Dancing a merry jig will also improve your mood.

...before exercise

Good carbs and some protein are the best things to eat, so wholemeal pasta with a bit of chicken would be good. Houmous and avocado wholemeal sandwiches will sort you out too.

...after exercise

Something high in protein with a balance of high and low glycaemic carbs. Bananas are perfect for instant energy, as are nuts, raisins and fruit smoothies. And plenty of water, of course.

...when you are on an average high street

A good chicken kebab is OK – lean grilled chicken, with lots of salad and some bread isn't a bad meal choice. Fresh green salads and wholemeal sandwiches are good too, but stay away from stuff that's swimming in mayo and rubbery cheese.

...when you are out on a big date

Avoid Jerusalem artichokes, known for their legendary wind-generating power. Traditional aphrodisiacs such as oysters are rich in zinc, which increases the male sperm count and thus is more useful later in the relationship.

What's all this about allergies and food intolerance?

We don't know if you've noticed, but more people than ever seem to be allergic to or 'intolerant' of certain types of food than ever before. This whole area is quite confusing, so we thought we'd try to make things a bit clearer.

Allergies are the most serious and involve the immune system, which will immediately reject the particular food as 'unsafe'. The immune system releases chemicals to combat the 'unsafe' food and thus causes an allergic reaction, leading to uncomfortable physical effects such as vomiting, swelling or a rash. Nice.

Then there's food intolerance. People sometimes have bad reactions to foods that don't involve the immune system, but can still cause discomfort. The effects may not be apparent for hours or even days, which can make diagnosis tricky.

And there's food 'aversion'. This can just be down to the fact that people don't like a certain food, and once they know they have consumed it, they may have a bad reaction, not unlike the reaction to an intolerance. What is interesting here is that if the person doesn't know they have consumed the particular food, they are unlikely to have such a reaction, from which you can infer that it is not initially a physical problem.

The bottom line is that if you have an allergic reaction (an immediate reaction to a certain food) then see your GP. And if you think you have an intolerance, then also have a word with your doctor.

But don't self-diagnose. There is an increasing tendency for people to decide for themselves that they are wheat intolerant after eating four thick doorstep sandwiches and feeling a bit bloated. If in doubt, always ask an expert – speak to a doctor or qualified nutritional expert, and don't start cutting important things out of your diet because you 'might' be intolerant.

Booze – will it make me look cool?

Erm, not really*. And it's not that good for you either, but that doesn't stop people from enjoying a few pints of bitter shandy after a hard day's stapling. So we thought we'd outline our four-point booze-management system (BMS), which enables you to stay on speaking terms with your liver.

1 Eat before drinking. This slows down absorption into your bloodstream, making you less likely to be the first person up to do karaoke.

2 Drink a glass of water for every glass of booze. Rehydrating as you go along will stave off the bad effects the morning after.

3 Drink yourself healthy with fresh fruit juice mixers, which contain antioxidants to help combat the bad stuff in the booze.

4 If you've drunk too much, stay off the sauce for at least 48 hours afterwards to give your liver time to clear out the rubbish.

*Unless you're drinking Campari.

So how much can you drink?*

Government guidelines suggest that women can drink up to
2 to 3 units a day and men up to 3 to 4 units a day, without
significant risk to their health. And you can't save them all up
for the weekend.

A unit of alcohol equals...

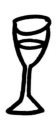
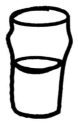

A small glass
of wine

Half a pint of normal
strength lager

A pub measure
of a spirit

*This is not a challenge.

So what we're saying is...

1 vary your diet so you're getting plenty of everything – carbs, proteins and good fats

2 try to get more low glycaemic index foods into your everyday intake

3 make a decent packed lunch and share it with unhealthy friends

3a there is no magic solution – diets that omit whole food groups from your life are rubbish and unhealthy

It's time to do some exercise

But please don't put the book down now.

We're going to make it easy. We're going to make it so easy that you won't even think you're doing it. We're going to blend it into your day so that it isn't a chore. You get the idea.

Funny thing is, we thought about it and remembered that exercise is all about running, jumping, skipping, climbing and rolling around – things that actually sound enjoyable and natural, like mucking about in the park and throwing a ball around.

We've split exercise up into three areas of physical-ness:

- Aerobic – exercises that are all about getting you out of breath, getting your heart rate up and generally giving the most important muscle in your body a kick up the backside.

- Resistance – this is all about gently developing muscles, which will give you more energy and may tone your body to boot.

- Flexibility – or stretching to give it a more simple name. Being flexible will keep you relaxed, prevent muscles from stiffening and lessen the chances of muscle injury.

And we also look at some ideas for exercising your mind at the end of the book, so you'll be able to achieve Zen-like calmness on really hot sticky days when your bus is late.

One final thing – if you suffer from any health problems or are a bit unsure as to whether you should do any of our exercises, check with your doctor first. We can't be held responsible for any injuries, even chipped fingernails, and your GP knows best.

do some aerobic exercise

What is aerobic exercise?

Aerobic exercise is the stuff that increases your heartbeat and leaves you breathless and a bit sweaty; things like running and cycling. On top of all this, it also burns off excess fat, leaving you less lardy than before.

Evidence shows that regular aerobic exercise can reduce the risk of stroke and heart attack by 50%, reduce the risk of diabetes and improve the way our brains work. So definitely worth doing if you want to stay clever and fit (as opposed to slow and wheezy).

How much aerobic exercise should I do?

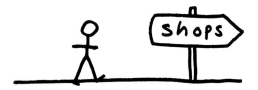

In an ideal world, we should all be doing three or four sessions of 30/40 minutes a week i.e. the equivalent of you not watching *EastEnders*. But the honest truth is that this is easier said than done.

So to help you we've done two things. Firstly, we've suggested some ways to make 'proper' aerobic exercise a bit easier to do. And secondly, for when you just aren't able to do the proper stuff, we've come up with some ways to make your average day a bit more aerobic, leaving you free to catch the omnibus on Sunday.

But what if I'm really lazy?

Well, you could do worse than filling out the contract below:

The innocent exercise contract

We, the lazy people, being of relatively sound body and mind, promise to…

(tick as many options as you like)

☐ run three laps of the park twice a week
☐ cycle to work three days a week
☐ do the weekly exercise schedule at the back of this book for the next six months

We understand that if we break this agreement, we are liable to…

☐ pay £75.00 to all other counter-signees
☐ do everyone's laundry and washing-up for the next three months
☐ wear flip-flops at all times next January

We agree that we can only opt out of this contract by producing a genuine doctor's note, thus excusing us from the agreed activities.

my name	signature	date
friend 1	signature	date
friend 2	signature	date
friend 3	signature	date

Get properly aerobic

No prizes for working out the best ways to get aerobically fit.
Allow us to suggest some ways to make them a bit easier to do.

Swimming

Gym

A few lengths will help to improve muscle definition as well as stimulate your ticker, and you may even get to see some nice people in their swimwear. To make it a bit easier...

- Organise a lunchtime swimming club at work. Mild peer pressure works wonders, and you can have races and everything.

- Don't get involved in any bombing or heavy petting.

The gym is quite expensive and everyone there is fitter than you. But it works a treat if you can be bothered to go. To make it a bit easier...

- Join with a friend who will encourage/humiliate you into going.

- Do exercise classes – more sociable and less boring than the treadmill.

- Get the gym people to draw you up a programme with some goals to aim for.

Running

The grandaddy of all aerobic exercise. But start slowly – too much too soon will increase the risk of injury. Begin on grass (much easier on the joints) and run short distances at first. The right level of exertion should mean you are still able to have a conversation with someone and not be too out of breath. To make it a bit easier...

- Have a target e.g. train for a 10km fun run (it will be fun, honest).

- Join a running club.

- Find a partner to run with who also likes the idea of wearing a towelling headband.

Cycling

Cycling is cool, especially if you can do wheelies. And they always say that cyclists are the fittest people around, so it would seem like a good thing to do. To make it a bit easier...

- Pedal to work three days a week and knock your weekly aerobic quota on the head.

- At the weekend, cycle to the nearest country pub, where you can refuel on shandy and a cheese ploughman's.

Check www.sustrans.org.uk for cycle routes all over the UK.

What aerobic stuff can I work into an average day?

OK. We accept that not everyone is going to go running three times a week. So here are some clever and unclever ways to do aerobic things all day. The bottom line is that it's your heart, so only you can really keep it healthy, but doing these things will help, promise.

Walk more

Sit on the top deck of the bus, take the stairs not the lift, use the photocopier on the next floor, walk to work and don't crawl anywhere.

Dancing

Dancing gets you out of breath, so join a class and amaze the boy/girl of your dreams with your salsa moves or headspins.

Clean the house

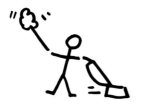

Vigorous hoovering, dusting, window-cleaning and bath-scrubbing are the bomb when it comes to exercising your heart, as the cool kids might say.

The shopping trip

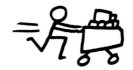

Leave the car at home, stick a rucksack on your back and a shopping list in your pocket. Briskly walk or jog to the supermarket, purchase goods and walk home laden with your stuff at a pace that generates a light sweat.

Get off the bus

Get off one or two stops early and walk the rest of the way to work.

Kiss chase

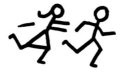

Ever since man lived in caves, he has brightened up the day with a quick game of kiss chase. So do what comes naturally.

What we reckon

We don't want to get all heavy or anything, but it's worth saying that every bit of aerobic exercise you do will help you to extend the length and quality of the life you're living. And unless you are a firm believer in coming back next time as a chihuahua, this is pretty much the only chance you'll get.

We're not saying you can't carry on eating crisps and watching *When Pets Do House Makeovers* when you get home. But make sure you've done something aerobic during the day so that your heart doesn't go looking for a new owner.

In conclusion...

1. do something aerobic today, even if it's just a fast walk to the shops

2. set a target with a friend, so that in 6 months you're doing laps of the park with ease

3. play kiss chase every single day of your life

resistance is not futile

What is resistance exercise?

Resistance exercise is the stuff that makes your body look nice and toned, and it's achieved by getting your skeletal muscles to do a bit more work than usual. Traditionally this is done with the aid of weights, but it's worth pointing out that the aim here is not to turn you into Mr T.

Resistance training has a whole host of other benefits such as helping to improve your balance and increase your metabolism (meaning that fats gets burned quicker) as well as giving your muscles nice definition and shape, rather than making them bulge through your t-shirt. And your attractive new physique will increase the chances of you being linked with Jenny Lopez/ Duncan out of Blue on the gossip pages.

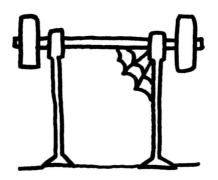

Will resistance exercises turn my beer belly into muscles?

In a word, no. Fat and muscle are completely different things and don't 'turn into' one another. Exercise burns fat and tones muscles, so a good all-round exercise programme will burn your fat belly away, meaning that you'll now actually be able to see the six-pack that has been hidden for so long. Staying off the Mars bars will help as well.

How much do you need to do?

It all depends on how buff you want to be. If you're like us, you'll probably be happy with just looking healthy rather than developing strange new muscles. So an exercise should consist of 'sets' of five to eight repetitions of a certain movement.

Start off nice and easy, doing lots of different exercises but just one set of each. Then make incremental increases once you can handle what you're doing comfortably, one set at a time. And change your routine so your body doesn't get too used to them.

You also need to rest lots. What you are essentially doing is damaging your muscles so that they'll repair themselves and get a bit stronger each time. So take a couple of days off every 3-4 weeks, and make sure that you eat well and get lots of sleep – your body does most of its repairing when you are snoozing.

Some important words about your back

The exercises that follow are as safe as houses, but before you start doing them, please make sure you're being kind to your back. Everyone knows you shouldn't lift with your back – what you need to do instead is maintain a 'neutral spine', which basically means a little bit of a curve in your lower back, with your bum out (not too far) and your chest out. Brace your trunk in a way that feels like you are stopping yourself having a wee and then see if your belly button moves back about half an inch and keep braced. Now you're in neutral and ready to go. NB Please don't be scared of the floating skull. It's not real.

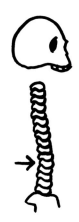

Why should I bother?

If you spend most of the day on the sofa, you'll start to lack muscular strength, making physical tasks a bit more strenuous and stressful. The more these tasks tax our bodies, the more we tend to avoid doing them, contributing to a downward spiral in our muscular health. So break the habit and do some of the stuff on the next few pages.

What can I do that doesn't involve joining a gym?

Don't get us wrong – we like going to the gym (sort of). But if you want to read about gym-based resistance training, we are sure that there are better books elsewhere in the shops.

What we want to do is give you resistance exercises you can do at home/down the youth club/in the middle of a large department store on a Saturday afternoon. So that's what you'll find on the following pages. The exercises are split into things you can do by yourself ('solo cabine', as the French might say) and those that you can do with a friend.

Good luck, and look after your back.

Stuff you can do by yourself

Toilet squats

Aim to keep your chest up and bottom out (quite literally). Sit back slowly, touch the seat and then come slowly back up. It's important to keep your body weight on your heels – don't rest on the seat – and put your arms out in front of you for balance. Five reps should do the trick. Great for toned legs.

Fred Astaire stairs

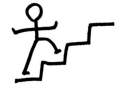

Find lots of stairs. Then run up them whilst moving from side to side like in those old movies. You can continue to change position as you go up and get fancy with your footwork. Great for the legs but also brilliant for balance and your bum. Do it till you just can't dance no more.

Door holds

Stand against the door frame, keeping your spine in neutral and pressed against the frame. Then bend your legs, lowering yourself, keeping your heels on the ground. When you're as low as is comfortable, hold the position and feel the burn. The length of time you hold and the depth you go is purely up to you – the longer and deeper you go, the harder it gets. A certified 'nice thighs' exercise.

Heavy pies

Before putting them into the oven, use your pies as weights and do a set or two of pie-lifts. Your reward, of course, is that you get to eat all the pies. And you get toned arm muscles as well.

TV heaven

(Or how to sort out your bum and stomach whilst watching *Lovejoy*.)

Beginner

Lie on the sofa with most of your back on it, legs out in front. Squeeze your bum until you are capable of lifting your hips to form a straight line with your upper body. Hold for 30-60 seconds and repeat five times.

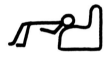

Intermediate

Move yourself down the sofa so that only your shoulders and head are in contact. Think about that stopping-a-pee-feeling in your stomach. Squeeze your bum and make your belly button sink just a little without dropping your hips. Hold as above. Build up to five reps, holding for a minute each time.

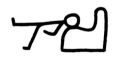

BAFTA-award-winning

Raise one leg off the floor, pushing your weight off the floor with your standing leg. Squeeze your bum hard on that side, and make sure your hip doesn't drop. Keep shoulders, hips and raised leg level. Start at five times, 30 seconds each side, and build up to 1 minute.

Bin lifts

Pen pick-ups

Put a pen on the floor in front of you. Balance on one leg and keep your chest up and bum out. Start to take the free leg backwards and once you're as far back as possible, you'll need to bend the supporting leg to keep your back in the right position. Pick up your pen, push back up and repeat. Remember to change legs. If you're not that flexible, start with a cereal packet and then move on to a football (intermediate) before attempting the pen. Magic for your legs.

The difficulty lies in how heavy you make the bin, so start with an empty one. Hold the bin at chest height and squat down (chest up, bum out, weight on heels). On your way back up, push the bin above your head. Repeat five times for nice healthy shoulders and arms.

Bath time

A pretty tough one to end with. Hold onto each side of the bath, taking the strain in the shoulders and arms, and lift your legs and lower body up and out of the bath water. The closer your knees are to you, the easier it is; when you get stronger, straighten your legs a little and take more time getting in and out. An advanced version is to lift your bum and legs up out of the water and then slowly swing your legs out over the side of the bath. Works wonders for your stomach.

One leg chair squats

Put the top of one foot on a chair with the other leg out in front. Lower your body, keeping a neutral spine and bending your front leg. Swap legs. The deeper you go, the harder it will be and the bigger the stretch on your legs. Great for overall body stability as well as your legs.

Stuff you can do with with a friend

Wrestling

Whether on the floor or standing up, this is one of the best exercises that you can do – it'll train your entire body, particularly your stomach. Start off with some light wrestling, maybe with your gran, before moving on to more taxing opponents. Variations on this theme include Love Wrestling with that special someone, and Office Wrestling, to sort out disputes in lengthy meetings.

Moving house

Please don't buy a new house just to do this, but if you hear of any friends who are moving, offer to help. They may buy you a gift for all of your hard work.

Girl/Boyfriend lift

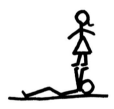

Lie on the floor and ask your partner to step onto your hands, which should be vertically above your shoulders in a bench-pressing position. Then try to lift them. This is quite a tricky one, and should only be attempted if you can do all of the other exercises in this section. And if you have full medical insurance.

Plank off

Go head to head with a partner. Both of you should assume the plank position (a bit like the raised bit of a press-up, but resting on your elbows and lower arms, which should be flat on the ground, instead of on your hands). The plank is great for your stomach – you should see who can stay in the position for longest before collapsing.

What we reckon

Well, we reckon of all of the bits of the book, this is the bit you're least likely to want to get involved in. It's the bit that feels most like work. But let us just say again – if you don't train your muscles, they won't use energy efficiently, meaning you'll get tired and chubby. And you don't need to do loads – 15 minutes a day is a start...

In conclusion...

1 you don't need to join a gym to do resistance exercises

2 doing resistance exercises will make you look nice and toned without turning you into Van Damme

3 we're not joking about wrestling

be
flexible

What does flexibility mean?

Flexibility often gets overlooked in favour of 'proper' exercises like running, lifting, etc. Which is a shame, as without a bit of stretching, muscles can get bunched up, rather than attractively giving your body tone and definition. Being flexible also improves your posture, meaning that you lessen the chance of suffering from back problems. And it just feels good – what beats a good stretch after a long nap on the sofa?

So we advise you try to build some flexibility into your average day, either by doing one of the activities described overleaf, or by doing some of our simple exercises, which come later on in this section.

How do I stretch properly?

You should aim to slowly move into a position of 'mild discomfort' ('ooh' rather than 'ouch') when stretching. Hold the stretch for 10-30 secs and allow three to four repetitions for each.

Organised flexibility

There are a few ways to stretch in an organised fashion i.e. with other people, doing some sort of activity that is based around staying flexible. Two of our favourites are yoga and capoeira.

Yoga

Yoga is basically a set of prescribed stretches. Of course, there are many deeper and more mystical meanings to it, but fundamentally its aim is to keep you flexible.

Its image has changed from the mung bean/leotard-based ones formed by people in the 1970s. Nowadays, yoga classes are full of nice, normal (and attractive) people, and for some of the class you get to lie on the floor, listening to plinky-plonk music while inhaling incense, which can't be bad.

For more info, check the British Wheel of Yoga at www.bwy.org.uk

Capoeira

Capoeira is that sort-of-dancing that looks a bit like slowed down karate. Its place of origin is unclear (Africa? Portugal?) but it is thought to have been started by slaves, who were trying to hide their fighting techniques with music and dance.

Ultimately, capoeira is a contact sport, but it is largely practised as more of a playful art, and its beauty lies within the strength and agility needed to become a good capoeirista.

When learning capoeira, you have to memorize set moves, as you would when learning judo or a certain dance, and through carrying out combinations of moves, your muscles are flexed and stretched.

Check out www.capoeirauk.co.uk
and www.londonschoolofcapoeira.co.uk for more.

Being flexible on an average day

Coming up are some easy stretches that you can do wherever you happen to be during the day. But you should look to stay active and flexible all of the time; don't slump in your swivel chair all day. If you want to get really serious, set a reminder to go off every hour or two that tells you to get up and have a five-minute stretch. And meetings can get pretty boring, so suggest a two-minute stretch before you begin. Seeing the boss touching his/her toes is always worth it.

Warming up and warming down

Experts now believe that the traditional warm up (lots of funny groin and hamstring stretches) isn't necessary. Your warm up should use moves that gently replicate the activity you're about to do, which kind of makes sense. Warming down is more important – it reduces the shortening of muscles that occurs during exercise, and stops lactic acid from building up, meaning that you won't be as stiff in the morning.

Coffee table stretch

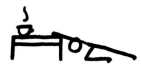

Make a square position with your arms, body and legs while kneeling on the floor with a low table in front of you. Place your hands on the table and make a straight line with your arms and back. You will feel the stretch under the armpits. Once in this position, concentrate on gently pushing your chest forward. If you want to stretch more, move your knees back, but don't move so far that it starts to hurt.

One-legged hoovering

This will stretch the back of the legs, and you should feel the muscles in your bum working too. Stretch right out to get to those difficult to clean bits; to do this you may need to bend the supporting leg. Try not to bend your back by keeping your chest out.

Snake hips

Put the top of one foot behind you onto the seat of a chair. This leg will now be in a V shape. You will feel a stretch through the front of the leg running into your hips. Push the hips forward to increase the stretch. For added snakeness, make a hissing sound and flick your tongue in and out rapidly.

Star maker

Lie on the floor and place your arms above your head and stretch for the wall behind you. Concentrate on making yourself as tall as possible through your upper body. Turn your feet so that the insteps try to touch the floor. While doing this, work on keeping the shoulders down. A great overall body stretch.

In doors

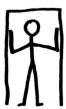

Using the door frame, lift your arms out at right angles and place them with your forearms resting vertically on the door frame. Push your chest out a little, keep your shoulder blades down and back. Move forward to increase the stretch.

The lunge

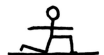

Take a step forward, then bend the back leg. Move slowly into the movement and emphasise the weight of your body being pushed through the hips. You will feel a stretch on the front of the back leg and hip and the back of the opposite lower leg. Make sure you keep your trunk upright and your front heel in contact with the floor.

Reach for the sky

Cradle rocking

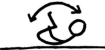

This one is amazing for your back.
Lie on your back with your hands
under your knees. Draw your knees
up to your chest or as far as is comfortable. Roll gently back and forward. You will be able to roll further
as you relax more but don't roll any
further than your shoulders. Go side
to side for a variation on the above.

Stand up straight and stretch your
arms above your head. Keep your
arms in line with your ears and keep
your palms touching, reaching as far
as you can upwards. You should feel
your stomach muscles stretching.
Bend your legs slightly, pushing your
weight onto your heels whilst maintaining the position above. You won't
be able to lower yourself more than a
few inches, but you'll definitely feel the
power of this stretch.

What we reckon

It's difficult to get away from the fact that these days we lead more sedentary lives than ever, so even if you just get up a few times a day and spend five minutes stretching, you'll be keeping your body awake and your muscles strong. And you should feel more relaxed too – stretching and flexing is a great way to keep your mind calm.

So please be bendy.

So what we're saying is...

1 don't skip stretching – it means you'll be less likely to get injured doing other things

2 get up from your desk every hour and have a stretch

3 be like the blade of grass that bends in the wind, rather than the tall oak that breaks in the storm*

*wax on, wax off

mind yourself

And relax...

Our minds get enough exercise. From dusk till dawn, they're full of thoughts, decisions to be made and problems to be solved. So finding time to relax and to empty your head of its everyday garbage is of the utmost importance.

What we've also realised is that the health of your mind is connected to everything else in this book. If you have a balanced diet and do a bit of exercise, your brain will be fuelled, stimulated, and ready to solve sums such as 1345 + 2478*.

Of course, there will still be times when you lose it or get stressed or upset. We can't come round to cheer you up when you're sad (though we'll try if you give us a ring on +44 20 8600 3939). But we can try to give you a few ideas to help keep your mind in good working order, and to help you relax when the world has been hassling you for even more stuff than usual. We hope you find them useful.

*=3822

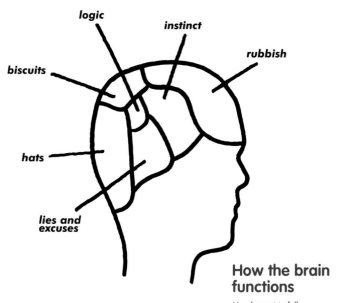

logic

instinct

rubbish

biscuits

hats

lies and
excuses

How the brain functions

Man has yet to fully understand the workings of this complex machine

Keep your brain healthy

It's funny – people spend loads of time on their six-packs and biceps, but they don't really think about their brains in the same way. Which is a shame.

Without going over the top, you carry nature's greatest miracle around with you every day. Just the fact that you're reading this and understanding the words puts every computer on the planet to shame. Your brain can make more connections and patterns of thought than there are atoms in the universe, and to top it all, it remembers complicated plot-lines in *Coronation Street*.

So here are a few ways in which you can keep it in shape:

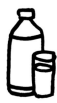

Your brain is mainly made up of water. Even a small amount of dehydration will stop it from working properly, so drink your 2 litres every day.

Your brain needs a steady, reliable source of fuel, so eat good carbs that don't mess up your blood sugar levels.

B vitamins help to manage depression and also increase the efficiency of your memory and concentration span. Get good B vitamins from fish, soya (tofu etc), greens, raisins, pumpkin seeds, eggs, brown rice, oats and chicken.

A quick walk round the block will increase your intake of oxygen and keep your brain fuelled.

Give your brain a break

Your brain has done a lot for you over the years. It helped you in that spelling test back in primary school, and it invented a very good excuse to get you out of trouble when the chemistry lab burned down. But what have you ever done in return?

We suggest treating your brain to small holidays whenever possible, so it can rest and recharge.

- Never eat lunch at your desk – it's the devil's work. Give yourself a full hour at lunchtime to go to the park, or find a quiet place to sit and have a cup of tea.

- Unplug your TV one evening a week and do something else.

- Have a nap. It's been proven that a snooze at lunchtime will mean that you'll be more awake in the afternoon.

- Have a warm bath when you get in from work. Opening the window and staring at the sky, even if you can only see a little bit of it, will help you feel nice and calm whilst having a soak.

Have a brain-friendly weekend

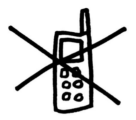

Instead of doing the same old rubbish, spend a weekend being
kind to your mind. Eat the right stuff (see page 133), take
a couple of quiet walks in the park, read your favourite book,
listen to some relaxing music, avoid the pub and go to bed
at 11pm.

Don't watch films or read newspapers and turn your phone off.
The world will still be there when you get back. Even if you only
do this once in a while, you'll find that Monday morning is a
whole different place.

Calm calm calm

Meditation is simply the art of concentrating on the natural rhythm of your breathing and allowing your brain to have a rest. So it's the ultimate lazy exercise – no movement, no thinking, just breathing. Now, before your head fills with images of levitating yogis, we'd like to say that we have meditated on the bus, at work and even in the pub (once). It's easy and you don't need henna tattoos to do it – just start off with three basic steps:

1 Ideally, wear something comfortable. Tight jeans and pointy fashion shoes can be discarded at this point.

2 Set your posture – sit in a comfortable position with a straight back (resting against a wall might help). Let the rest of your body hang freely around your nice straight back.

3 Relax thoroughly. Close your eyes, start taking deep breaths and loosen the muscles in the face, neck, arms and hands. Do a mental check, starting at the top of your head and moving down through the body, making sure that all muscles are relaxed.

Once you are fully relaxed and breathing slowly and deeply, just concentrate on the rhythm of your breathing. It might help if you also picture one specific thing that takes you away from the everyday e.g. your favourite place. Keep doing this until your mind feels calm and empty, before slowly opening your eyes and returning to real life. Even five minutes will make a difference, promise.

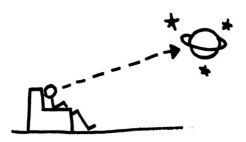

One of our favourite ways to start meditating is to imagine floating above our very own Fruit Towers. Gently rising, our field of vision increases, taking in beautiful Shepherds Bush, then west London, then the UK, etc, etc, until we are looking down on the Earth and leaving the atmosphere, moving further out into space. If you are reading this in space, then try it the opposite way round.

In a nutshell

1 when your brain is tired give it a rest; even a 5 minute nap is better than nothing

2 drink lots of water to keep your brain working properly

3 call us if your brain stops working and we'll send you the office spare

An innocent exercise routine

As recommended by us...

Monday

Get off the bus p.95

Door holds p.106

Reach for the sky p.124

Tuesday

Toilet squats p.105

The lunge p.123

Swimming p.92

Wednesday

One-legged
Hoovering p.121

Shopping trip p.95

Heavy pies p.106

Thursday

Running p.93

Coffee table stretch p.121

Fred Astaire stairs p.105

Friday

Cycling p.93

Cradle rocking p.124

TV heaven p.107

At the weekend

Bath time p.109

Kiss chase p.95

Sleep

It's a flexible schedule – swap other exercises in and out as you wish. The most important thing is not to think of exercise as a chore, and to start doing a little every day. Because the more little bits you do, the happier and fitter you'll be.

Thanks for making it to the end of the week

If everything's gone to plan, it should be seven days since you read the first section, and you will have learned a few new things to help you stay a bit more healthy.

But of course, there's nothing new under the sun. Most of the stuff in this book is common sense; the basics of staying healthy that most people are aware of. The tricky bit is doing it, but hopefully we've given you enough tips to make this a bit easier.

Our ultimate hope is that you incorporate a few of our ideas into your average day. We're not asking you to bench press Shetland ponies or run a marathon in two hours – we just want you to stay alive a bit longer because, well, it would be sad to lose you just because you couldn't be bothered to get out of your swivel chair/Japanese sports car to walk to the shops once in a while.

So we'll see you around – in the park, on your bike or maybe down the pub drinking a hard-earned cup of beer after doing that exercise where you watch telly whilst staying fit*.

Bye for now.

*Page 107 in case you're interested.

We did this

Words and one of the pictures – Dan Germain
Design and all but one of the pictures – Joby Barnard
Exercises and dietary advice – Pete Williams at Health Dept www.healthdept.co.uk
Nutritional consultant – Professor Joe Millward PhD DSc RPHNutr
Watchful eye – Richard Reed

Thanks to

…everyone at innocent for their help, encouragement and recipes (sorry if we didn't use yours)…Ingrid Connell and Gordon Wise at Boxtree for waiting patiently…Pete and all at Health Dept for teaching us about exercise…Nigel Slater, Fiona Ruane, Yvonne Foran, Jessica's mum, Steve (Assia's boyfriend), Zach, lovely Clare, Kylie, Lucy E, Lucy T, Brontë, Nina, Jessica…Cardigan Bay's very own David Hieatt www.howies.co.uk…Professor Joe Millward for always making sure things are right…all of the people who drink our drinks and get in touch with us. Please keep doing it at stayhealthybelazy@innocentdrinks.co.uk

Acknowledgements

Appetite - Nigel Slater (Fourth Estate, 2001) – p.50
And we'd like to acknowledge the fact that the sum on p.130 is wrong.

Books that helped us while we were writing this one

Fitness for Life Manual - Matt Roberts (Dorling Kindersley, 2002)
The Food Doctor - Ian Marber (Collins & Brown, 1999)
The Oxford Book of Health Foods - J G Vaughan & P A Judd (OUP, 2003)
The Oxford Companion to Food - Alan Davidson (OUP, 1999)
Winning Ways with Cheese - Mary Berry (Purnell, 1983)